I'm Just Like You

m.e. Elzey

Published by Little House Press, 2025.

I'M JUST LIKE YOU

First edition. March 10, 2025.

Copyright © 2025 m.e. Elzey.

ISBN: 978-1734054682

Written by m.e. Elzey.

Dedication

To all the selfless heroes who have given all they had to help those who struggle with a facial difference. The unsung heroes who created support groups around the world. They have gone to extraordinary lengths to ensure everyone with a facial difference knows they are not alone. Working to make sure that everyone has a seat at the table and to insure no one ever feels alone. We are lucky to have them fighting for our future.

"This is the true joy in life, being used for a purpose recognized by yourself as a mighty one. Being a force of nature instead of a feverish, selfish little clod of ailments and grievances, complaining that the world will not devote itself to making you happy. I am of the opinion that my life belongs to the whole community and as long as I live, it is my privilege to do for it what I can. I want to be thoroughly used up when I die, for the harder I work, the more I live. I rejoice in life for its own sake. Life is no brief candle to me. It is a sort of splendid torch which I have got hold of for the moment and I want to make it burn as brightly as possible before handing it on to future generations."

George Bernard Shaw

Prologue

A friend advised me to only focus on the psychosocial aspects of living with a facial difference. Stay in your own lane. Broadening the focus of this essay would be too much.

Another friend advised to do the opposite and make the essay's theme about bigotry as the common thread between all marginalized people. I'm all too familiar with discrimination toward my face. My wife of 52 years is a Mexican American and for her entire life has been she's been the focus of racial and ethnic slurs. Doing my small part in making a difference about how we treat each other. My hope is by sharing my story and beliefs, it will make a difference. I want the readers of this essay to understand the toll it takes for those of us who are the focus of discrimination regardless of their difference.

This essay is about sharing how I lived my life with a facial difference. It is as much about how I perceived myself as how others saw me. I must confess, despite others' discrimination against me, I inflicted a lot of wounds upon myself.

I hope people will read this short essay. Some of you will be relieved to find that you can relate to many of my experiences. With a bit of luck, others will notice the issues, visible and invisible, confronting many people. My hope is you will reconsider your stereotypes about those of us with a facial difference, or any disability. Maybe someday, when you meet someone with a different appearance, you will not look twice at their face. Or perhaps you will reconsider before requesting another table when the restaurant host/hostess sits you at a table next to a person with a facial difference. Maybe you will be a little more understanding of those who are different regardless of the reason. Become less judgmental. Start challenging what's acceptable in a so-called normal appearance.

What matters is not my deeds, but the instances where I encountered bias based on my appearance. I did not need to stand out in the crowd. My face garnered much more attention than I wanted.

Marginalized people need to be reminded that their lives matter. I share how I lived my life with the damage bulbar polio inflicted on my face. Some readers connect with what I have lived through. Perhaps by sharing my experiences and beliefs will make a difference for people, like me. People who do not fit in. I hope my story will give a little solace to the parents of a child who is different for any reason.

From early childhood, I have lived my life with the disfiguring aftermath of bulbar polio, diagnosed on July 5, 1951. The day ranked among the worst of my parents' lives.

To me, the most devastating consequence of bulbar polio was survival itself. In my youth, I suffered terrible bouts of depression. Even questioning why, I should bother wanting to continue to live.

Now that I am an old man; I like my face. This provided a unique understanding of human nature, encompassing both its capacity for cruelty and kindness. This provided a chance to examine many personal convictions. My conviction is that living with a facial difference made me a more considerate person.

Bigotry is the core issue in my story. The misguided bigotry of my youth, and the prejudice of people and institutions, had an impact. Humans concoct all kinds of pseudo-legitimate reasons to justify our fear of those among us who are different, whether real or imagined. Clinging to our core prejudices for dear life, even though we forgot the reason for our own bigotry. Most of us are rather comfortable with the way we view the world. We are certain of the logic behind our bigoted beliefs.

I did not carry a notebook around with me during my life. Some stories are my best recollection of events that happened many years ago. These stories and events defined who I became as an adult. My personal story shows the joys I experienced during my life and the unexpected pleasures I felt along the way.

I shared personal reflections that most influenced my life. I challenged long-held beliefs by many institutions that discourage inclusion.

We codified our fears and bigotry as city ordinances, religious dogma, or political rhetoric. No matter how we try to improve the appearance, this is unapologetic bigotry. How can we make any change if we hold bigoted ideas about who gets full access to opportunities? How do we bring about change in a society where many do not see the need?

As a Baby Boomer, I grew up in rural Arizona during the fifties and sixties. I started my life having snow-white hair, bright blue eyes, and almost translucent skin. If I was born a decade earlier in Nazi Germany, I might have been a poster child for the Third Reich. However, if I contracted bulbar polio in Germany under the Nazis, their Aktion T4 (eugenics) would have ended my life for not living up to the expectations of the supposed superiority of the Arian race.

I find imagining the experiences of women, racial minorities, homeless individuals, and gay people difficult. I am not mentally ill, neither am I an immigrant farm worker living in the shadows of California's Central Valley. The difficulties some people go through for the basic necessities of life is far beyond my ability to comprehend.

I have learned a few things in my life. People stared, and many eateries refused to serve me. My distinct facial features have resulted in mockery, marginalization, ostracism, and bullying from others. Experiencing this bigotry gets tiresome.

Count me out with people or organizations with values that discriminate against others. Allowing for prejudice to maintain a friendship will not happen.

The snake-oil salesperson possesses the answers to the most pressing issues of our era. Those who say they know everything are the con artist.

The United States marginalized indigenous peoples. We enslaved African people and dehumanized them long after their enslavement ended. We never liked immigrants and treated them with nothing but contempt, but we still profess to be a nation of immigrants.

Things become more chaotic. As strange as it may sound, across the United States for 100 years, cities implemented regulations that kept those with facial difference, people who look like me, out of sight. These last "ugly laws" ordinances disappeared from the books in 1974 in Omaha, Nebraska.

The United States also experienced race-centered city ordinances that became known as "sundown laws." Many city limits signs warned inferior races and repulsive looking people not to be caught within the city limits after dark!

Human history is full of actions that are abhorrent. If you are reading a country's or institutions' history and you are not wincing in disgust every now and again, you are not reading history; you are reading propaganda.

Notes

Throughout the writing and rewriting of this essay, I fluctuated on the most accurate term for people of my likeness. When I was a child, my family, doctors, and most others described my facial features as disfigured. Everything in life changes and so does our need to better define who we are. We are human beings with a facial differences caused by many kinds of maladies. Throughout this autobiographical essay, I use the term facial difference, not only because it defines who we are as people, but moreover because it is the right thing to do.

Please note that I changed the circumstances and the names of some stories to conceal their identities. I took a literary license to clarify some conversations. Remembering the precise points of a specific discussion is not possible, but how it affected me was crystal clear.

Included in the addendum of this essay is information you may find useful. The Faces ~ National Craniofacial Association has compiled a comprehensive list of a worldwide list of Support Groups, Camps and Retreats, and Educational Scholarships. I have included a link for you to access.

There is also a link to an abstract titled, "A hidden community: Facial disfigurement as a globally neglected human rights issue." Coauthored by Phyllida Swift and Kathleen Bogart. I encourage you to read this incredible abstract. The instructions on how to access the abstract is in the addendum. If you are interested in learning more about various aspects of disabilities, I added a short list of books. More information is available in the addendum.

My Family

I was born in San Fernando, California on February 7, 1950, to Kenneth Raymond Elzey and Leona Lucille Graham. I am the youngest of three sons, Kenneth Lee, my eldest brother. Darrel Raymond, no I did not misspell Darrel, our mother did, and me ... Mark Elwood.

My parents grew up in different parts of our country. My mother grew up in North Hollywood, California. Her stepfather worked in the motion picture industry.

My mother's biological father abandoned my grandmother prior to my mother's birth in Phoenix, Arizona, in 1922. After my mom's birth, her mother's family left Phoenix for better opportunities in Los Angeles. My mother was three years old when my grandmother married a man who worked in the movie industry. Her mother and stepfather's heavy drinking led to my grandmother being killed in an alcohol-related traffic accident in 1937, when my mother was fifteen.

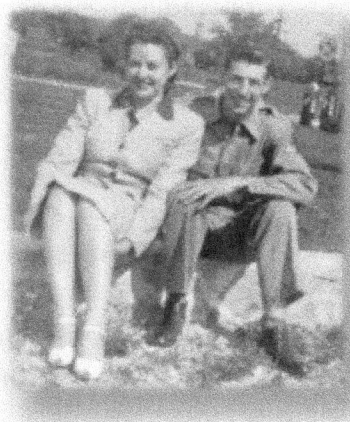

My father hailed from Milan, Illinois. He was skilled at storytelling. Employing Lincoln's wit and aphorisms to make points, and sometimes to annoy, was his style. Among my most cherished recollections is hearing my father recount his Illinois childhood. He was the son of the Mercer County roads superintendent and part-time farmer of a small patch of farmland. In 1935, his mother died of pneumonia. My father's life became even more difficult when my grandfather died in 1937, three weeks before my father's high school graduation. My dad was the sweetest, most humble man I ever knew. He remains my hero. I would deem myself successful if I someday achieved half his stature. The entire country was in the depths of the Great Depression. it mattered little where anyone lived. Everyone was struggling. The brutal economics of the times influenced their lives.

As if my parents' misfortunes were not enough, on December 7, 1941, the Japanese bombed Pearl Harbor without warning. America found itself on the precipice of the Second World War. Along with millions of other young men, my father joined the Army. My father served with honors as a First Lieutenant in Patten's Third Army. He seldom discussed his experiences.

On July 4, 1951, I was just like any seventeen-month-old child in America. By the end of the next day, I would be in the Los Angeles County Hospital Polio Isolation Ward withstanding an open tracheotomy, paralyzed and breathing with the help of an iron lung, where I spent the next two years of my young life. This one event would forever alter the trajectory of our lives.

My mother left my brothers with a neighbor and took me to the emergency room of San Fernando hospital. When I arrived at the hospital, my back arched backwards, and I became unconscious. As the day progressed, my entire body became paralyzed. A doctor told my parents I either contracted Meningitis or Poliomyelitis and planned to transport me to Los Angeles County Hospital.

I cannot imagine what my parents experienced after the doctors diagnosed me with bulbar polio. I spent three of my first five years in the polio ward. That is a long stay for anyone at any age. The period is especially lengthy during the initial five years of life. This is an important time, especially for children, because ninety percent of brain growth happens between birth and five years old. I understand we are born with all of our brain cells. Brain growth refers to the millions upon millions of connections a child's brain makes every day. This is a crucial period for the growth of social skills, cognitive abilities, language skills, and social-emotional development.

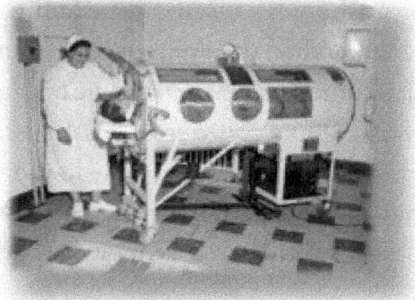

My first recollection is of seeing the mirror over my head fixed to the iron lung. I remember the beige color paint on the walls. I remember the location of the swinging doors, where my iron lung lay in relation to others in the room, and the Black nurse who cared for me. The nurses would move us from time to time. They moved my iron lung next to a window overlooking a parking lot. I looked through the overhead mirror, out the window, and down to the sparkling wet parking lot. Rain fell as people rushed to and from their vehicles. I am unaware of the polio isolation ward's location, but the rain on the people in that wet parking lot remains vivid in my memory.

A few weeks before my planned hospital discharge, the physicians asked to meet with my parents. At that meeting, the doctors proposed to my parents that I be raised in an institution. Their assessment was that it would be easier for me to be with other children experiencing similar conditions. They stressed that it would be simpler for my parents, my brothers, and especially for me. My parents did not need to think about their suggestion. They responded to the doctors with a resounding NO!

One of the last conversations with my mother before her death concerned an event I vaguely recalled. At six years old, I had been out of the hospital for about two years. We were all getting dressed up as a family for an outing. I remember my older brother Darrel fastening my belt while we were standing in the doorway to our small San Fernando home. I recall standing in the driveway of a man who lived at the end of the small block next door to friends of my parents, Rose and Pinky. Yes... their real names, scout's honor!

Pinky noticed his next-door neighbor washing his car and me standing at the end of his neighbor's driveway. He watched the event unfold from his kitchen window. The neighbor yelled something at me, then he began drenching me with water from the hose. Pinky ran out of his house, yelling at him. I remember Pinky picking me up and carrying me home.

My mother filled in the gaps of what happened that day, in August 1956. Pinky's breath left him speechless. He told my parents what had happened.

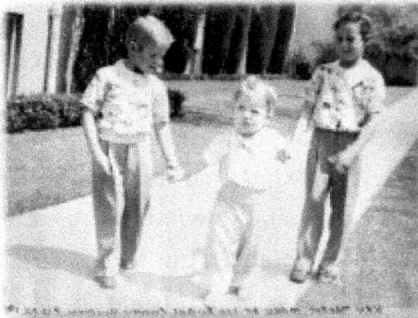

He was livid and set on confronting the neighbor who sprayed me with the water hose. Pinky, a man in his early sixties with a prosthetic leg, intervened and convinced my dad to let the police take care of the neighbor.

My mother said Rose, Pinky's wife, called the police. She began berating the man, daring him to spray her with the hose. Everyone in the neighborhood heard Rose's barking voice. Pinky, concerned Rose would escalate the matter, returned home to defuse the situation. After the police arrived, my father calmed down. The neighbor claimed the event was accidental. My mother explained that without Pinky's presence to defuse the situation, things could have concluded otherwise.

The events of that August afternoon will remain uncertain. That situation so upset my parents that they sold our home by October. Our family moved to a little agricultural/railroad town twenty-five miles southeast of Phoenix, named Gilbert, Arizona.

I was six years old when we reached our new residence at 502 South Catalina Street on Columbus Day 1956.

Cowboys, Cattle, and Cotton

The small country town of Gilbert differed from today's suburban bedroom community. In 1956 it was an idyllic small Western town famous for the alfalfa and cotton grown on the surrounding farms. The small town was along the Southern Pacific railroad line. Gilbert was a southwestern copy of a Norman Rockwell painting, only with cowboys, cattle, and cotton.

Even before we left San Fernando to live in Gilbert, I knew how people responded to my acquired facial difference. Those reactions ranged from kind and understanding to repulsed at the sight of me. To this day, whenever I go out in public, someone always seems obliged to take a second look at my face.

As a seven-year-old, I wanted friends. My seven-year-old self-concluded that by being funny relieved some of their tension, my face provoked. As a child, I received much compassion after surviving bulbar polio. The virus caused the deaths of many children afflicted with this terrible disease. Being the youngest and no doubt a little spoiled, I exploited the situation to the best of my abilities. I was funny when all I wanted to do was to connect with other children, hoping they would disregard my facial difference.

I started Gilbert Elementary in the first grade. Most of the bigotry directed toward me by kids and adults alike came as polite avoidance. Blatant prejudice seldom appeared, but this occurred enough for me to become a master of hiding my genuine feelings.

My seven-year-old self's only wish involved entering a room without attracting attention. Perhaps someday people would not notice me. I would be just another face in the crowd, enjoying the moment with friends. That dream never came true. My whole life, I was the subject of stares and gossip. A few people made it clear that my facial difference was not welcome.

The questions, gossip, and stares of some classmates proved difficult. Bigotry from grownups caused more pain. Mrs. Hall, my third grade elementary school teacher, believed I had a cognitive impairment. I stood in line for lunch when I unintentionally spat on a classmate (one of the many aftereffects of bulbar polio is an excessive amount of saliva that I produced). The kid got upset and told Mrs. Hall, who got angry at me and sent me to the principal's office. I decided I had had enough of Mrs. Hall and school. I went home, enough was enough.

That incident came to a climax when my parents insisted on having a private meeting with Mrs. Hall and the principal. The meeting ended after Mrs. Hall informed my parents; I disrupted the other students. She explained I made many of the kids uncomfortable around me.

As if Mrs. Hall had not said enough, she continued. I lacked normal intelligence. She continued by telling my parents that a child like me deterred the other children from learning. She insisted I should be with kids like me. My father, the most mild-mannered man in the world, stood up to address the teacher. The principal stood between my father and the teacher. That evening, the principal came to our home to apologize. That was when, for the first time, an adult showed such careful consideration of my facial difference.

Prior to high school, I envisioned following in the footsteps of my two older brothers. I intended to be an outstanding student, an above average athlete, and most of all, I would be popular. My high school experience was unlike my expectations. I became preoccupied with self-pity.

The starkest difference between my brother's high school experiences was that I emotionally checked out before my freshman year. My grades were mediocre at best. Sports remained impossible because of my left arm and hand atrophy and neck paralysis. Regarding popularity, I had too little time for anything else but nonconformity. Through all of my high school years, I did not attend a single sporting event. I pretended high school mattered little to me. Yet deep down inside, in a place I kept to myself. I would have done anything to be accepted. Looking back at the way I acted in high school; I do not know how did my mom and dad put up with me?

This story does not reflect their parenting skills. As an adult, I recall how my parents handled a situation about my high school senior photograph. My parents insisted a photographer who specialized in photo touch-ups take my photo. After being told me about their plans, I responded by telling them I did not want my senior class photo taken at all. They insisted, and under protest, I complied.

A few weeks later, an "airbrushed" version of the face my parents wanted to see came in the mail. The altered photograph is their ideal of me, not the way I looked. My parents confirmed my face fell short of their approval. My face being different was the only thing my parents and I agreed on. I find reviewing their choice difficult, even after all this time. That is how things were, and I can only describe my emotions with certainty. If my appearance wasn't good enough for my parents, how did others react? Concerning my appearance, the elephant in the room was a major topic of avoidance, especially if I was present.

The image did not depict me. The photo only confirmed the photographer's airbrushing skills. After seeing the photograph, it meant nothing to me. Thirty-some years later, following the deaths of both my parents, the airbrushed photo was meaningless to me as I threw it away.

Had one of my daughters had a facial anomaly, I would do everything in my power to prepare her for the inevitable. Instilling in them it is okay being different, regardless of the reason. We will love you regardless. No strings attached. There would be no doubt I would love and accept them the way they are.

I had no idea how to navigate high school. By creating a world full of barriers, I dealt with it the only way I knew how. No one would ever know the real vulnerable me. I did not confide in anyone, neither family nor friends. The scars from bulbar polio was my issue, not theirs. I would not let myself become anyone's charity case!

I have only one life, and when it is over, it is over. Why am I burdened with such an unattractive face? I hated my face, and I resented the stares and gawking that came with it. The stares, the snickers, and being one of those weirdoes who did not fit in made me resentful.

I did not realize at the time nor did my parents, but if I had seen a psychotherapist, I would have learned better coping skills to use. I believe it would have calmed my nerves. If my child was different for any reason, they would receive counseling, not to "cure" anything but to help them develop much needed coping skills from a cruel public. I learned my coping skills in my forties during a year of counseling.

Over the years, despite all the bumps and grinds, I have grown to like my face, even the parts that do not work. I reached my forties before I realized my face, although banged up by life, looked just fine and dandy. If only I had realized that years sooner. Please do not waste time with self-pity!

The Incident at the Walk-In Theater

I clung to the popular beliefs of the day, attitudes that defined most everyone's place in our society. Beliefs that dictated the roles we played in our society in the mid-twentieth century. Minorities, women, and the disabled had a specific, immutable stature. I would soon learn that society did not accept me.

I felt America's history had hit rock bottom. We lived in constant fear of the domino effect of communism that would spread around the globe. Our soldiers risked their lives in Vietnam, protesters at home demanded we get out of the war.

Black people insisted on having equal rights. I thought Martin Luther King was a communist stirring rebellion among Black people. If black people did not like it here, they were welcome to leave anytime! Immigrants had the audacity to start a union for farm workers that guaranteed better working conditions. Black people, Latino people, women, hippies, and homosexuals wanted a piece of the pie.

One evening in August 1967, in just a couple of minutes, my entire worldview would forever change. I traveled alone to see the released film "Bonnie and Clyde," playing at the Mesa Theater ten miles north of Gilbert. I was standing in line to buy a ticket when this guy behind me walked around to get a better look at my face. After a thorough examination, he burst out laughing. I ignored him, as I always did in those situations. He returned to his place in line behind me and soon after; started insisting I tell him what happened to my face. Maybe he was showing off to his girlfriend when he inquired about what happened, using more vulgar language. I ignored his questions and taunts again. Even though I was in front of him, his voice and language showed growing irritation. Without warning, from behind, he struck me with his open hand, slapped me on top of my right ear. I have been largely deaf in my right ear since that evening. The force of his strike knocked me to the concrete.

"Do I have your attention?" he shouted.

After getting back on my feet, I saw his pure, undiluted hatred for me. Why did he hate me so much because of my face? Did he intend to kill me? People reacting violently toward me had happened before, but never with such intensity. I knew, without a doubt, that I was all alone when the other people in line scattered. Tears streamed down my face while I covered my ear and looked at him. I felt the blood running between my fingers and down my right arm.

"What the hell happened to your ugly ass, f**ked up face?"

After I got back up, he slapped me as hard as he could across the left side of my face. Again, slamming me down to the concrete.

I wore braces. The force of his second slap embedded the braces into the tissue of my left cheek. People scattered out of the way while I again got up from the concrete. I did not keep track of the time, but everything happened so fast. I do not remember what happened to him. All I knew for sure is that he was gone. No one in the crowd bothered to help me. I walked to my dad's truck and drove through the countryside back to Gilbert.

Halfway back to Gilbert, when the pain in my mouth became excruciating, I parked in the darkness along a dirt road near an irrigation ditch. Using my finger, I dislodged the metal braces inside my left cheek, which hurt a lot, and bled even more. The pain and the reminder that I was different and not wanted made me sob. That night underscored what I had known my entire life, but never admitted. I would never belong, regardless of how hard I tried.

Sitting in the cab of my dad's truck for an hour before driving back home on the dirt country roads that surrounded Gilbert in the Sixties. I arrived home that evening around midnight. My parents were in bed but not asleep. I said hello and went to the bathroom. I cleaned the remaining blood from my right ear and face, then took three pain pills. The swelling on my left cheek caught my attention. I was going through nonstop facial reconstruction surgeries and procedures.

The next morning, my dad noted that my cheek looked swollen and asked if it hurt. I told him a little. It is because of the work doctors were doing on my palate.

That brief encounter at the theater changed my life. The unprovoked attack because of my facial difference shook me to my core. Over time, this incident, among others, caused me to reexamine some of my fundamental beliefs. It would be one of the many violent acts directed at me because of my facial difference.

To this day, I do not know who the guy was. I kept that event to myself until I told my wife many years after that evening.

So why do I tell you this story? The reaction to my face has brought out the best and the worst in people. Why did he hit me? What did I do? How did I offend him? All these years later, I wonder if he remembers me? All I have is questions and no answers. After that night, I have paid close attention to my surroundings.

Crippled Children's Hospital Phoenix, Arizona

My parents and I visited a plastic surgeon in Phoenix. After he examined my face, he told us he could repair the bone structure and some of the tissue, however he could not correct the damage from the paralysis cause by bulbar polio. The left side of my face and the upper left side of my body would remain paralyzed.

I turned fifteen in the spring of 1965 and, with a lot of kids that age, I lived in a whirlwind of contradictions. The process began when a team of doctors started planning to fix the harm bulbar polio caused to my face.

I recall wishing above all to look like everyone else, with all the components of my face and upper body functioning. I felt about the medical procedures necessary for achieving that goal. The most troublesome part involved realizing the entire purpose aimed to improve my appearance, not to cause offense.

From a cosmetic perspective, the facial damage bulbar polio caused was extensive. Paralysis of the seventh cranial nerve caused the left side of my face to droop. In comparison, the drooping skin presented a less significant problem than the damaged bone structure. My face may not have looked functional, but I got by. I enunciated words well enough for people to understand me, despite a slight nasal resonance in my voice.

I hoped, once the doctors finished, I would be normal. People would never stare at me again. All the issues that came with a facial difference would be gone forever.

On one level, I was eager to have the surgeries, which would allow me to live a "normal" existence. On another level, I resented having to go through the pain of reconstruction surgeries and procedures just to be easier on the eye. My bitterness grew as the doctors worked through my high school years to reconstruct my face.

My parents learned their health insurance would not cover the cost of reconstructing my face. According to my parents, when I first contracted bulbar polio, the taxpayers of California paid the tab for the years I spent in the hospital in Los Angeles, over a million dollars in 1950s money. Fifteen years later, the doctors, the hospital, and all the accompanying expenses were compliments of the taxpayers of Arizona, another million over a four-year period, 1965 through 1969. Every Christmas vacation and summer break starting in the eighth grade through high school, I spent in the hospital for major surgery. I have a lot of outpatient procedures, some causing pain for months at a time.

I did not tell my classmates or the few friends I had about the operations. Had I told them about my surgeries and no one came to visit, it would have devastated me. Except for my parents, I saw no one, and that suited me just fine.

I fantasized I would go back to school after one of these surgeries, looking normal. Everyone would admire the astonishing difference the surgery made and they would see just how handsome I was. After every surgery, my face looked like I was in the boxing ring with Mohammed Ali. The swelling, bruising, and pain took a long time to disappear.

Doctors extracted my wisdom teeth early so my jaw could mend before its reconstruction. Within months of my wisdom teeth extraction, orthodontists fitted me with braces to align my upper and lower teeth. My palate, which was also disfigured from polio, also needed to be reconstructed.

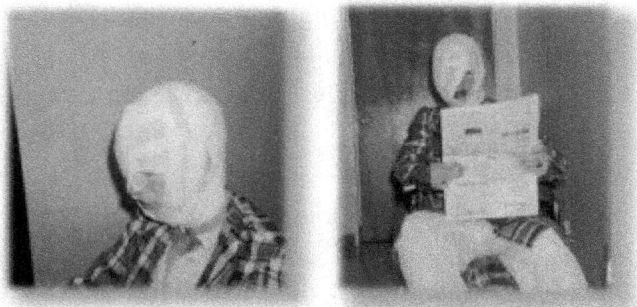

The doctors slowly cracked the upper hard tissue of my palate and moved my left cheek bone out where it should have been. This procedure was the root cause of a six-month never-ending headache. After my bone structure was in place but not healed, the doctors did a facelift on the left side, the drooped side of my face. They used fascia from the upper part of my right leg. Fascia is the elastic tissue that surrounds our muscles.

After the facelift doctors operated on the thin tissue around my left eye. Doctors have operated on my left eye eleven times. The last surgery was when I was seventy years old.

In May 1968, four years after doctors started repairing the facial damage from bulbar polio, they rebuilt my mandible. Surgeons reshaped my jaw in a seven-hour operation, then wired my jaw shut for the following four months. There were 80 dissolvable stitches inside my mouth and the same number outside my jawline on my neck.

What did all this rebuilding of my face do to me? I learned surgeries do not help me feel better about myself. All those years ago, I did not realize no doctor — then or now—had the power to improve my attitude toward my situation.

Becoming someone who mattered was a decision I alone had to make. Whether different in appearance, the ability to choose is ours alone. The responsibility fell to me to grow up and get past my ego. Everyone has bad things that happen to them. If you expect to always being treated fairly, you are on the wrong planet.

My parents showed amazing support throughout the entire effort to improve my life. I had a chip on my shoulder and resented having to go through all the procedures and surgeries. As a teenager, I vented my frustrations on my parents by causing them a never-ending series of problems.

In retrospect, throughout my difficult adolescence, I questioned my parents' steadfastness. I lacked experience and understanding of the world in my youth. I did not yet realize the world was not created to make me happy.

My last surgery was a minor operation during Christmas vacation of 1968. My facial reconstruction concluded when I had reached my fill. I told my parents if people did not like the way I looked, they should turn their heads. I graduated from Gilbert High School the following May and, with that, my childhood ended. It was time to get on with the rest of my life.

Even after four years of reconstruction surgery, I did not view my facial difference favorably. Two childhood friends lost their lives in Vietnam. My life's trajectory further fueled my disillusionment. My frustrated, caring father reminded me that unlike the two kids from Gilbert who lost their lives in Vietnam, I still could change if I would stop the whining and grow up!

Jeannie

The story of the rest of my life began at the Union 76 gas station in Gilbert. I was filling my 1971 orange Volkswagen bug. I was minding my own business when a beautiful Mexican girl pulled up in a 1957 turquoise Chevrolet. Gilbert was a small town when we met. I knew of her, but not well. One thing led to another. The following Friday marked our first date.

Fifty-three years have passed since then. Today, we have two beautiful daughters and five wonderful grandchildren. We had our challenges. She remains my north star.

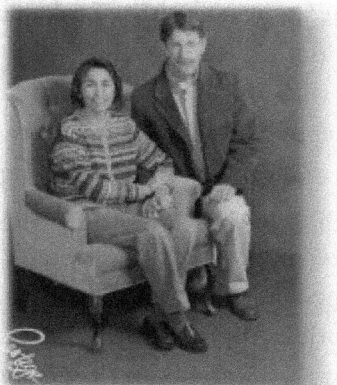

Jeannie (Juanita is her given name) is a Mexican-American gal and not so faithful Catholic. I am a non-religious white kid. Our small conservative town frowned upon inter-ethnic dating.

My parents were caring, loving people whose values I hold dear to this day. Most white Americans of that era assigned minorities' specific positions in society. Black or Mexican people should never have lived in our neighborhood, much less begin dating their children...but they did.

Most of the white adults familiar to me during my Arizona childhood subscribed to the soft bigotry of low expectations toward Mexicans. The primary and secondary education of the time reflected those same values. My parents' and their generation's view of the world differed from today, however bigotry is far from a thing of the past.

What connection does this brief history lesson possess to a tale regarding my face? The answer is, everything about our societal attitudes toward minorities, the role of women, the disabled, and individuals with my similar appearance.

I had a facial difference. How could I be a bigot? Me being a racist or a bigot was unimaginable. I was so enlightened, but only in my mind. Not having the ability to recognize my racist actions of telling ethnic jokes and not being aware of the impact. She would ask me again and again to not tell those jokes. I told her many times she was too sensitive. I told her to lighten up. It was a joke! What harm could it cause?

A relative of mine told a joke about a guy with a cleft lip and palate. I did not see the humor. I also noticed she kept looking at me out of the corner of her eye as she told the joke. On the way home that evening, Jeannie asked me about my experience being the brunt of a joke. "That represented the classless, crude jokes you told about ethnicity," she said.

Having to swallow some of my own medicine is the worst taste imaginable. People tell crude, tasteless stories only to belittle others. Jokes slurring the disabled or a racial minority say more about the person telling them than anything else. Whether the individuals sharing these narratives are clueless or indifferent is unimportant. Stories that belittle people are wrong.

We are all raised with ideas about the proper values to espouse. We learn role modeling from our parents while other behavior we collect along the way. Certain beliefs proved commendable, while others fell short. I harbored all kinds of stereotypical ideas about Mexican Americans when I first met Jeannie. I was unaware of my prejudice, but it was there. Prejudice shaped my understanding of Mexicans. We are more like other humans on this planet than we care to admit. We must learn how to be more compassionate along the way.

I questioned others' opinions of those similar to me. Yet deep down in the dark places where reality lives, the answer to the question was already clear to me. My desire to be a 'normal' looking person was so misguided I ignored the almost daily reminders. I questioned my development of this idea of superiority over others. Somehow, I realized I had become one of those crude, repulsive people I despised. No different from those who gawk at me when I am out in public. I made it the goal of my life to change how I viewed others, the world, and myself. This all happened because of Jeannie.

I get annoyed when I hear people complain about being "woke" or having to be correct in their social interactions. They complain some people will be offended. We need to be more aware of how our words and actions affect others. If it means conforming to accepted standards of conduct, then so be it! We cannot complain about the way people respond to our faces and yet turn around and belittle others for their differences.

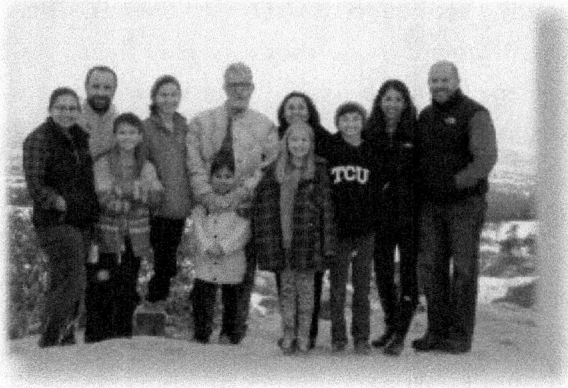

Jeannie and I got married, and soon after, our daughter Maria arrived. Three years later, we had another daughter, Lisa. While my wife was pregnant with both daughters, I was worried that our child would be born with some kind of facial anomaly. I couldn't bear the thought of my children going through what I went through growing up. I was so worried I barely slept through my wife's entire pregnancy. On the day Maria was born, I was ill with worry. When the nurse brought her to the window for me to see, all I looked at was her little face. Not noticing the nurse's big smile and the fact she pulled back the blanket so I could see her entire little body. My intense focus on her facial features caused me to ignore everything else. I asked the nurse if our baby was okay. She answered, "Your daughter is perfect, although banged up a little from being born." The relief was enormous, that I cried. I felt the same way when our second daughter was born. They remain, and always have been, the most perfect daughters anyone could envision.

Young people asked about my wife and my story. Our worldviews showed considerable discrepancies. From the beginning, we agreed to be equal partners committed to making our marriage last.

Along with other adult mentors, I talked to various young people with facial differences over the past forty years. During our conversations, we discussed romance and finding acceptance for their differences. This is a normal concern. They want someone who they can share their lives. I felt the same worries as a teenager in the sixties. I met my wife, and we both worked hard to make our marriage last. On January 6, 2025, we celebrated our 52nd anniversary. We faced many challenges throughout the years, but we overcame them and persevered.

The Yin and Yang of Working Life

Motorola Semiconductor Products Sector had over twenty thousand individuals within our Motorola division. With that many people, you will find just the person you are looking for... and some of them will find you.

Most people I encountered during my 34 years at Motorola showed honesty and a strong work ethic, showing no interest, one way or the other, in my facial difference. To my coworkers, the only thing that mattered to them was: did I fulfill my work related responsibility? As usual, some individuals had significant problems with my facial difference. This small but outspoken group of people who found my appearance offensive. Perhaps they thought I disfigured my face just to piss them off. They made extraordinary efforts to keep me away from them. I cannot control if a person likes or dislikes me for whatever reason.

The vignettes I write about in this section are people who impacted my career and my outlook on life. Some taught me how to handle troublesome people. Others set an example through their grace and demeanor. These people inspired me throughout my career and my life.

I have been fortunate. A former supervisor said, "It's amazing how lucky you get when you work your rear off!"

This section is about how I managed a successful career with a facial difference. This concerns the people encountered throughout my professional life. I am so thankful for my years of Motorola employment. Few companies existed in the Phoenix area to offer jobs during the late 1960s and early 1970s. My dad worked for Air Research, a company who built gas turbine engines. They also did not hire relatives of employees. My two older brothers and I could not work for Air Research. Motorola Semiconductor Products Sector represented another option. My oldest brother Ken started in 1964 and retired in 2008 for a forty-four-year career. My other brother Darrel started in 1966 and quit in less than a month. It was not his cup of tea!

Thanks for my brother Ken's help. I started in 1972 and had a thirty-four-year career. Upon starting at Motorola, I only sought employment. There was no all-encompassing lifelong plan. I lacked any degree to ready myself for a corporate job in electronics. Even though I was a junior at Arizona State University, burnout overwhelmed me. I was young and clueless about what I needed to know. I suspect I am not the only young person in this difficult situation. Young and naive about the ways of the world, I trudged ahead.

I am proud to say that for thirty-four years I worked for the Motorola Semiconductor Products Sector (SPS) of Motorola Communications a maker of car phones, walky-talkies, two-way radios, flip phones, and a plethora of other electronic communication devices used around the globe.

My lifelong professional affiliation lay with the division producing discrete semiconductors, digital large scale integrated circuits, linear integrated circuits, digital signal processors, microprocessors, and microcomputers.

Our division took the lead over all other electronic component manufacturers on Earth in redefining communications. The industry introduced technology, enabling electronic communication devices to send messages globally in nanoseconds (operating speeds measured in billionths of a second, the speed of light). Someday soon, modern state-of-the-art devices will operate in Pico-seconds (speeds that are measured in trillions of a second). The world is indeed changing. I am proud to have played a minor role in introducing our world changing technology to customers.

Motorola's division alone employed twenty-two thousand people worldwide. We worked with and developed some of the most sophisticated equipment ever devised by people. That era witnessed unprecedented innovation spanning numerous sectors. Select high-tech tools came about because of solid-state devices developed and produced by Motorola and several other businesses. I began my career in 1972 and retired in 2006. I encountered and collaborated with extraordinary individuals across the globe, representing varied life experiences.

It did not go unnoticed that I was in an industry producing the most intricate human-made products ever made, yet amid this brilliance there were some who found my looks appalling. We live in a crazy world.

Mike

An opportunities bulletin board showed a job opening as a production control analyst. Even though I had only worked at Motorola for just over a year, I decided I would apply to see what happened. The following is how I remember my first internal, within Motorola, job interview.

I am awaiting the guy who is supposed to interview me when he walked into his small office cubical. He glanced at me, acknowledged me, put some papers on his desk, and left without a word. I heard him speaking to his administrative assistant just outside the cubical.

"Is this a joke?" he asked the woman sitting outside his office.

"I'm sorry?" she responded.

"The guy in my office. Is someone being funny?"

"Not that I know of."

Silence followed. He came into his office and took a seat. "Hello, I'm Mike," wearing a shocked expression on his face.

"My name is Mark."

"So, Mark, you caught me off guard. What's going on with your face?" His finger making a circular motion around his own face, "Nobody said anything to me about your face."

"I had polio," I answered.

"Seriously? You had polio of the face?" He grinned. "That's a first."

At that point, I knew there was no chance of getting this job. "It was caused by bulbar polio a different type of polio than FDR contracted."

"Okay, I see," he responded. "Do you have any mental issues because of the way your face looks?"

"No, I don't think so," I answered, wondering to myself how this jerk got to be where he was.

We discussed different aspects of my face throughout the interview. How I got along with other people? We finished with the pretense of an interview in less than ten minutes. I thought it interesting that Mike didn't say a word about the requirements of the job.

The interview did not discourage me. I kept applying for a better job. Like most people, I failed more than succeeded. In other opportunities, I advanced because of my brother Ken's help; I took the new position without a second thought.

Hank

My boss assigned me to be on a task force. Because of my various commitments, I cannot remember why the meeting happened. By pure chance, someone mentioned the Americans with Disabilities Act (ADA) during a break and began discussing the legislation. I shared my limited knowledge; the law safeguarded those with visible differences.

Things went downhill fast. To my surprise, a quite unpretentious guy named Hank, whom I knew, or at least thought I knew for many years, got upset. Saying my understanding of the ADA was incorrect and the notion it shielded individuals who looked like me defied belief. After noticing my seriousness and likely correctness, he began grilling me about my feelings. I did not have an opinion because my focus on work prevented me from getting any significant understanding of the legislation. He believed my responses to his inquiries were condescending.

Hank got infuriated and mentioned my mother and my birth status. The situation deteriorated. He became so upset the person in charge of the meeting had to get involved in calming him down. Hank was so consumed with anger he did not attend the balance of the meeting. We were not friends, but I admired his perceived character from a distance. He never spoke to me again. To this day, I am still perplexed by the intensity of his reaction.

Motorola, like many other companies, would not employ me without my brother's help. It's doubtful I would have received many opportunities without his help. I am not putting myself down. It reflected the era more than company operations.

Getting a job is one thing. Maintaining the position and performing well is a separate matter. My goal was to be the best at every task the company gave me. I started my career as an inventory control clerk for small signal plastic discrete semiconductors. That is a lot to swallow! Discrete electronic components and integrated circuits preceded the microchips and microcomputers, forming the basis of modern electronics encompassing smart phones, personal computers, and millions of other devices that changed the entire world. My role when I left Motorola 34 years later, in April 2006, included Vice President Area Director of Midwestern Sales, managing 150 million in annual sales.

I got off to a poor start, but then again, being young and naive about the politics of moving up in the corporate world did not help. Along the way, I established some key contacts and also experienced major roadblocks. Perhaps not because of my facial difference, but because everyone faces challenges. I was no exception.

Richard & Karen

A chance encounter on a sidewalk - Saint Charles, Missouri

One afternoon, my wife and I sat at a sidewalk café in St. Charles, Missouri. I noticed a man and a woman staring at me and whispering to each other.

My initial reaction was, 'Ah geez, here we go again!'

The man approached. "Are you Mark Elzey?"

"Yeah," I answered. "Do I know you?"

"I don't think so. One evening after work, I heard you talk about Motorola's electronic components you sell."

I acknowledged what he said. He continued.

"I want you to understand my admiration for you." My older sister contracted Bell's Palsy and has not been out in public in almost a year. People's reaction to her face caused so much trauma that she refused to leave her house.

We discussed his sister's Bell's palsy and my bulbar polio for a few minutes. We invited the couple to join us for coffee, but they needed to meet friends.

"Are you aware of everyone you have motivated?" he asked me. "I told my sister about you and because of you she worked up the nerve to go out in public again."

What this man related to me on that St. Charles, Missouri sidewalk, made up some of the most valuable words anyone has ever spoken to me. The man complimenting me on that St. Charles sidewalk also did not care how I got the job. He cared about his sister and I inspired him to talk to her.

That chance encounter preoccupied my mind as I reflected on the afternoon's events. If the woman with Bell's Palsy had been the only person I ever inspired, that would have made all the ridiculous bigotry I put up with over the years worthwhile. I was certain that at least I made a minor difference in a person's life. If that is all I did, then I was a success!

In my career and life, I committed to doing what was required to succeed. It was a simple equation; failure would not happen, no matter what. The most important thing in my life was my wife Jeannie and our daughters. They were amazing, and I wanted to do everything possible to ensure our marriage lasted a lifetime.

A brief word about my brother Ken helping me advance my career at Motorola. Throughout my entire career I heard the claim that the only reason I got a promotion was because my brother helped me. Indeed, my brother helped me out a few times. It is the exact sentiment black people received who advanced in their careers, "*The only reason you got that job was because of equal opportunity laws,*" It was a bigoted statement when they made it to a black person. It was equally bigoted when people said it or worse implied it when they said it to me.

Let me share with you a story about Hattie McDaniel, a trail blazing African American actress, singer-songwriter, and comedian. When she landed the role of Mammy in Gone with the Wind, she was the first black actress to get a major movie role. Eighty-five years later. she still inspires African American actors in today's movie industry. They are enjoying their success in part because of the trail blazing accomplishments of Hattie McDaniel. She braved the storm of American racial bigotry and prospered!

Throughout my Motorola career, many people minimized my accomplishments. They credited my success to my brother's help. Not once did I ever deny his occasional help along the way. Getting a job is one thing, keeping it is a whole new ball game. I took the jobs knowing up front there would be comments, and there was! I didn't rest on my laurels. I worked hard to make sure I not only met the requirements of the job that I gave it all that I had. Who noticed? Richard, the man I met at the sidewalk café in St. Charles, Missouri, was the first person of many people to tell their stories. My promotion drew some criticism, but most people were thrilled. Oh yeah, you know who else noticed? Men and women who looked like me! That alone made putting up with all the bigotry worth it. I would do it all over again!

Geno

Being with Motorola for less than two weeks, I barely remembered where the restrooms were. I just entered the men's restroom when a disabled man leaving the restroom lost his balance. I was in the right place at the right time, so I grabbed him, preventing a nasty fall. It was pure happenstance.

Geno appreciated me being there to help him out. My impression was that he oversaw janitorial services. He wore normal unpretentious clothes and not the middle management standard dress during the 1970s, God-awful polyester sky blue bell-bottom pants, black patent leather shoes, with long sleeve shirts with extra-large collars and cuffs. Geno proved to be a decent, down-to-earth gentleman.

A few days later, during my break, while sitting on a bench smoking a cigarette, Geno joined me and we began talking. Without missing a beat, he reached over and took the pack of cigarettes out of my shirt pocket. He took one cigarette and put the pack back. I took my lighter out and lit his cigarette.

Calling him a friend would be inaccurate, but upon seeing him, I would greet him, and he would start a chat. I again had a smoke break when Geno sat down, began talking, and bummed a smoke.

At about that time, my supervisor Ray passed by and looked at me. Later that day, Ray came by the stockroom and asked if I knew Geno. I explained how Geno and I met and told Ray that I presumed he was a janitor or something similar. Ray told me that Geno was the second highest ranking manager in our entire division of Motorola.

Geno and I stayed in touch throughout my career. I cannot say we were friends, but we kept in touch with each other for many years. A short time after I went into sales for Motorola Semiconductors in Saint Louis,

Missouri, Geno called to congratulate me on my new assignment and wished me well. It meant the world to me he took the time to call.

Ray

I cannot imagine a better beginning than having a supervisor like my first boss, Ray. He remained an unassuming man from Pennsylvania, who took me under his wing and got my career off in a good direction. It bears repeating that getting an opportunity is only the first step; realizing its potential demanded considerable effort and devotion.

My aim became top performance in any role. There is no chance anyone would call me lazy or ungrateful for the chance. They could say I was young; I had a big mouth. They could say a lot of things, but they could not say I was lazy. I worked double hard and made it a point to do my job and to do it right.

Ray epitomized cool. I doubt I ever saw him come close to losing his temper. He belonged to those men who had a soothing impact on their companions. I always wanted to be like him, but I am just not wired that way.

One day, he visited the stockroom where I was working. I expected a severe reprimand regarding the conflict I had with another employee, but Ray's expression left me uncertain if anger was brewing within him. He kept thanking me for being such a hardworking and smart employee.

I felt bewildered, to put it mildly. With a breath taken, he looked me straight in the eye and told me I needed to grow up and resolve the problem with the other employee. He said that everyone was just trying to "make a buck" and it was hard enough without having to put up with an immature smart-ass kid. As he left, he made it a point to tell me once again how good I was. This is when I learned that the world did not revolve around me. I was a diligent, hard-working employee did not come with any form of privilege other than the opportunity to come back the next day and work.

Ray was my boss for the first two years. We remained friends for many years. When I think of decent, hard-working people, Ray was the benchmark for that position.

Pat

I knew Pat since I began at Motorola. The only thing I knew regarding her is that she is a lesbian. I wanted nothing to do with her. Not only that, she looked like the type of gal that had a serious edge. Her partner was Mary. They turned out to be the first openly gay couple I ever met.

I had been with Motorola for five years, and I worked in a department that included several special assignments. I arrived at work one morning to find my supervisor and his boss drinking coffee at my desk. This could have been a bad sign, but they appeared to be fine. My supervisor and his boss told me I'd been selected for a special project. They said the project would take six to nine months to finish. They explained the details of how I would do this task and said it would be a plus for my career, a feather in my hat, so to speak

Considering I did not have a choice, I accepted the assignment. No one in the department was available; my supervisors promised they would find someone to help.

Later that afternoon, I went to an off-site facility to get a first-hand view of the project details. A massive amount of work was awaiting me. Despite my supervisor's directions, I was uncertain how to fulfill their expectations. In the throes of a full-blown panic attack, the door opened, and Pat appeared. My initial reaction was, why is she here? I was not happy, but once again, I had little choice.

Pat proved to be one of the most thoughtful people I have ever known. She worked hard, and unselfishness marked her efforts to finish the job correctly and on schedule. We would eat lunch together, and soon we'd share stories about our lives. I discovered her parents and siblings had not been involved in her life for years. She said she always, even as a child, knew her sexual orientation.

Everything fell apart when Pat summoned the courage to tell her religious family. Her parents gave her an ultimatum to attend the gay conversion therapy through their church, or else.

Pat revealed her sexual orientation in the late 1950s. She spoke about who she is. Her parents, siblings, and church officials judged her as unworthy. She lost everything important to her for being honest. They took her religious beliefs and her strong family ties. The very foundation of everything she identified with.

I learned this assignment represented her only hope of staying at the company. Every supervisor gave a pseudo compelling reason to dismiss her from their department. She reached her limit. Her partner Mary sustained her. Both women radiated kindness and shared parallel narratives. Pat taught me grace comes in many forms and a person's character will carry them through tough times. I lost touch with Pat and Mary over the years, but I will always value what I learned from my friend Pat.

My venture into sales

After going into sales, some people did not hold back, insisting the sole reason for my employment stemmed from my brother, a fact I never denied. I secured a position unprecedented for someone with a comparable facial feature, as far as I am aware. Some took note and did not like me representing our company in sales! Their obsession with me going into sales did not bother me one little bit. They could hold their breath and stomp their feet for all I cared. I completed my necessary actions, regardless of how others felt.

In retrospect, I worked far too hard being in constant fear of losing my job because my facial difference made people uncomfortable. I regret working so extensively. When our daughters were young, I feared they endured taunts and teasing because of my appearance. Given the chance to restart my life, I would change my path. I failed to recognize my intense dedication to work to validate my presence. By working so hard,

I missed so much of what's important. I did not take the time to be with my wife and daughters because I worked too much trying to validate my existence. I was wrong. Don't make that mistake.

My point of view

In my junior year at Arizona State University, I killed a little time by going to a motivational speech by Leo Buscaglia, a public motivational speaker I had never heard of. I read his brochure on a bulletin board in front of Hayden Library. He sounded interesting, plus it was free. What a great deal! I sat on the left side of the auditorium about halfway up, in the smoking section! Yeah, I understand. How times have changed. His lecture's title: "The Art of Being Human." I listened to him. His lecture meant a lot to me. I existed in the middle period of my life. I was no longer a child, but I was not quite a grown-up either. Listening to him made me examine myself and how I interacted with others. This marked a fresh start, a novel approach to self-perception characterized by compassion. His last words that afternoon over 50 years ago stuck with me: "Never give advice. Smart people don't need it, and stupid people won't listen. Take care of yourself."

My greatest desire in my youth involved having friends. Throughout my memory, I could not find my place or be with those who wanted my friendship. To escape my reality, I started reading. Books kept me company. I also grew weary of people assuming a cognitive impairment based on my facial features. This motivated me to strive harder to show their mistake. The harder I tried to be accepted, the weirder I seemed to others. For a significant portion of my life, I experienced a continuous downward spiral of effort and failure, followed by further effort and failure. Why did I attempt friendship with those who refused to reciprocate? Yet I paid little attention to those who accepted me as I am. I am sharing this because I understand firsthand how hard life can be for people with a facial difference. I dealt with my difficulties in secret, as I had done in my youth. Please trust me, keeping your struggle to yourself is the worst thing you can do. Request help. Learn the skills to cope with difficult situations and troublesome people. We are born with a basic idea about life. After that, we learn everything, including how to respond to mistreatment by people or institutions. If you are unsure how to manage a situation, please seek professional guidance. I did. Counseling and learning coping skills made all the difference to me.

Relax, cool it, shake it off, breathe,
Be kind, it is as simple as that.
Don't give a second thought about what happened in your past
Or what may or may not happen in your future.
Don't let your life fritter away by worrying,
About the things you cannot change or control.
It's clutter! Don't get caught up in the minutia.
Don't get all fired up about what could have been,
What should have been.
Learn to accept everything for what it is.
You are only getting one chance to live your life to the fullest.
In life, there is no dress rehearsal.
Relax, cool it, shake it off, breathe.
Be where you are, in the moment, that is all there is.
Be kind especially to yourself. This moment is all we have.

m.e. Elzey

However you are different, you have the absolute right to be who you are, no matter what. Learn to like yourself just the way you are, regardless of what other people or institutions say.

Preventing people from participating has always been and will forever be a bad idea.

We are living in an era where old assumptions are being questioned. Are these assumptions still relevant? Did they ever matter? Some of these ideas formed the bedrock of our collective beliefs. Our world is struggling with dramatic changes never seen before in all of human history.

People are changing the concept of loving another human being. The LGBTQ community has fought a long hard battle for equal rights. Gay and transgendered people comprised a part of every society's makeup throughout history. Acknowledgment of their fundamental rights is long overdue.

We must demand basic human rights for all people, regardless of how society defines them. This new perspective has pressured religious institutions around the world. Religious beliefs that oppose gay marriage is nothing new. Sixty years ago, various religions used the exact argument against interracial marriage.

We used our religions to impose our ideas on how society should be. The Spanish Inquisition aptly shows a flawed concept's worsening trajectory. While Christopher meandered around the Atlantic looking for a different path to India, the Catholic Church under the direction of Pope Gregory attempted to change the dominate religions of the Iberian Peninsula, from Judaism and Islam to Roman Catholicism. The plan, AKA the Spanish Inquisition, started with a straightforward and simple question: "Do you want to live?" The rest is history. After Christopher Columbus blundered into Hispaniola, the authorities converted all the native peoples of North and South America. That effort is a permanent stain on human history.

Contemporary America has made progress toward racial equality over the past fifty years. That doesn't mean our work is done; we have much more to do. The pace of change is much too slow.

Perfection

The world was a mess on the day of our birth. It will be the same old muddled heap on the day we die. Our home is full of man-made problems of all shapes and sizes. That is how things are.

Today in the United States, over half of our population live in the suburbs, where all the houses are in a nice neat row lined with groomed yards. Homeowner associations keep a vigilant eye on our neighborhoods. They ensure all is perfect, preserving our idyllic scene. Neighborhood uniformity is important.

My wife and I live in the Tucson area. We have a medium size house with a nice desert landscape. Our communities take great care to groom the public areas. We watch television showcasing perfect-looking actors and go to the movies which feature even more perfect-looking actors. Everything is perfect.

The only thing is, this is an illusion. Most of us enjoy having order in our world. We feel uneasy when a yard's appearance deviates from the others on the block. We go to great lengths to ensure the "things" in our lives are how we want them. No space exists for anything different.

People are not things; they are sisters, brothers, aunts, uncles, moms, dads, daughters and sons. We cannot pick our relatives, race, ethnicity, gender or sexual orientation. In my life, I have discovered it's acceptable to be different.

We humans are always striving for perfection. Consider the case of Floyd Cochran. Floyd founded a white supremacist fanatical religion adhering to eugenics, a movement to eliminate undesirable people. That encompassed the Church of Jesus Christ and the Christian/Aryan Nations. Floyd resigned from the church after the other ranking members volunteered to euthanize his four-year-old son because of his genetic defect. Church scriptures he helped found stated his son's cleft palate and lip marked him as flawed in the eyes of their God. If you think this occurred a long time ago, you would be mistaken. That transpired in 1992.

This is an example, but in reality, people used religious dogma to justify racial prejudice, homophobia, and anything else you can imagine. If you have the itch to hate someone, or better yet, an entire group of people, claim their existence is immoral and forbidden, it even says so in the scriptures. Put on a condescending, disingenuous smile on your face and say, "It is not me; it is in the scriptures! We will love you no matter what. Followed by a subtle reminder that their beliefs are God's words, and disobedience will result in eternal damnation."

Some people have not fared well, securing a place at the table and enjoying life's abundance. We need to let go of our old divisive ideas about people. How can we ever expect to enjoy our lives if we take part in excluding others for an assortment of imaginary differences? Every person on this planet is fighting a tough battle. Despite our differences, everyone should be able to have a productive, meaningful life.

We need to facilitate future generations' pursuit of education, employment, and community belonging. By excluding others, how can we expect equal access? Buying into archaic ideas only doom all of us to permanent second-class status.

Exemplary behavior is one of our most vital actions. Showing a smile and being kind to others are examples of small but meaningful gestures. We need to stop being so judgmental. The small actions we perform each day create a significant impact. One person can change the outcome of many people's lives. We can offer hope to someone where none existed before. Sometimes having faith in yourself and your fellow humans is all that is necessary to make a remarkable difference. We each make daily choices that affect people in a positive or negative way.

Remember that wonderful experience when someone assisted you? Remember that sensation when you are out and about. Pay that feeling forward, because it matters. Don't overlook the people who came before you and gave hope in their own manner. We must do all we can to succeed, so the next generation will find things less challenging. To those with a facial difference who stay at home rather than face the public, please reconsider.

This essay is for those with facial differences. I shared experiences in my life so others in similar circumstances might relate. If for no other reason than to let people understand they are not alone. Polio paralyzed a facial nerve no bigger than a piece of butcher's twine, but the aftereffects preoccupied most my life. Revealing aspects of my life has proven challenging. Some memories came from the darkest recesses of my memories. Some memories will remain within me, far too difficult to share.

We are more than our facial differences. Similar to people worldwide, I exhibit positive attributes alongside flaws, a greater number than I will confess. We can draw conclusions about situations, or instead love and enjoy the essence of being human.

I know this seems paradoxical, but I assure you the statement is correct; Don't let fear hold you back from exploring the world or harboring resentment. Your life experiences surpass those of most others. These experiences give you a rare, important perspective on life. Don't wallow in self-pity.

User manuals explaining life with a facial difference don't exist. The experience of having a child or loved one with a distinguishing illness or condition is difficult to envision. We often offer help that is not wanted, which may leave everyone frustrated. One of the most difficult things in life is to understand what another person is going through.

Jeannie, my wife of fifty-two years, and I show an in-depth understanding of each other, yet we sometimes experience communication difficulties. Grasping and helping the people nearest to us—or who have been in our lives always—often escapes us.

A Casual Conversation

A colleague and I waited at the Oakland, California airport when a conversation started.

"I see you're taking next week off?"

"Yeah,"

"Going anywhere?"

"To a retreat."

"Oh yeah. What kind of retreat?"

"I'm one of three adult mentors to a bunch of teenagers."

"That doesn't sound like much fun. Is it a church group or something?"

"No, it's about fifteen kids and three adult mentors who come from all over the country."

"Good for you."

"The only problem is I'm supposed to be an adult mentor and I end up learning more about life than I contribute to these kids. They're so well-adjusted."

"I know the feeling. What brings everyone together?"

"We all have a facial difference. We hold these retreats from time to time for the kids to get together and share their experiences. It's incredible how these young people are so together; they're an impressive group of kids.

"Kind of a week-long group therapy thing?"

"Well, I suppose you could say that."

"Do you assist them in addressing their issues?"

"Oh sure."

"Like feelings of inferiority and stuff like that?"

"Excuse me? Wow, you caught me off guard. No, we don't do that."

"Why not?"

"I don't know, perhaps because this crossed none of our minds, or at least mine."

"Aren't you, kind of, skirting the issue?"

"What issue?"

"Inferiority complex?"

"What about that?"

"Why aren't you teaching these kids to deal with their inferiority complexes?"

"Like I said the kids have never mentioned the subject. I doubt any of these kids have this so-called inferiority complex. What makes you believe this is an issue?"

"Ah, come on, any person with a messed- up face has an inferiority complex."

"Oh yeah? Is that right?"

"I'm not trying to hurt your feelings but it's just common sense."

"Who knew? Do you think I have one of these inferiority complexes?"

"Well, since you brought it up, yeah."

We talked a while longer and you can guess where the conversation went from there. I decided I needed to get a book for the three-hour flight back home. I hoped the book would prevent further discussion about our mind-dulling conversation.

After that conversation at the Oakland Airport sparked my curiosity, I discussed the matter with the kids at the retreat. A few days later, the teenagers and I discussed feelings of inferiority. I posed the question to these kids, "Do any of you have feelings of inferiority?" Every child was self-conscious about their appearance. They had wholehearted support from family and friends.

In my forties, I sought guidance from a counselor to improve my ability to cope. We discussed a claim familiar to me for years. Acquaintances, friends, even some family assumed, because of my face, an inferiority complex afflicted me.

Sidewalk psychologists discussing inferiority complexes upset me. When I challenge this notion, the accuser's expression towards me implied not only inferiority but also a hint of insanity. People reaching that conclusion will never change their mind.

My counselor asked about my feelings of inadequacy. I responded no, but there were situations when I sensed inadequacy, but never inferiority. Perhaps some imagined how they would feel if their faces looked like mine? Would they have feelings of inferiority? One might assume if their faces resembled mine, they would harbor such feelings.

Once a family member told me that people did not stare at me, my imagination played a larger role than anything else. As people with any facial difference will tell you, people stare! Not everyone, mind you, only some are tacky enough to stare. This small group of people not only stare, but their rudeness is clear as they try to steal second and third glances at my face. Some show the audacity to point me out to their friends.

As a child, my parents instructed me to ignore those who stare and to dismiss those who make upsetting remarks. You remember the old saying, "Sticks and stones can break my bones but words can never hurt me." If you find yourself in a similar situation, leave as soon as possible. As with all people, situational awareness is always a good idea.

How often did you hear this: "Children can be so cruel!". Do children tease? Of course, they tease and they can be cruel, too. The minds of most children are full of an insatiable desire to explore and discover. Kids have not yet mastered the use of language. They just ask, "What happened to you?"

I was at a grocery store when a little boy looked up at me and asked what happened to my face. I smiled at him. Just as I was telling the little kid what happened, his mother flipped out! She was embarrassed and insisted her little boy apologize. I told the mother everything was fine; Adults are much more toxic in their reactions, sometimes disallowing children's curiosity. By the way, when a child is teasing, you can bet an adult is the one who taught the child.

When I mention this to people, some gaze at me in total disbelief, as if what I said could not be true. Today's adults are much better informed than a generation ago.

Zogby International

Zogby International has been tracking public opinion around the world since 1984. They conducted a poll for the "Game Show Network" called a "Report card on Prejudice in America". They polled over 10,000 people about matters of race, religion, political affiliation, and disabilities. Not only did they inquire about people's opinions on these topics, they reversed the questioning, asking the audience how everyone else in the group, plus others, viewed these issues. Search the Internet for the results of the entire report.

The following is verbatim from the "Report card on Prejudice in America":

On Disability: When asked to choose whom they believe most Americans would least want to work with, 26% of respondents said someone who is morbidly obese. Twenty-two percent said someone with a facial disfigurement. Respondents thought Americans would object much less to deaf (3%) and blind (1%) co-workers.

Americans offer acceptable responses when questioned on their own views about race and prejudice. That is why in this poll, we asked people about "most Americans'" views on race and prejudice. This provides a far more precise view of how people contemplate these matters. Americans are more forthcoming when discussing the problem in their neighbors' lives than in their own lives.

A little known history in cities across the United States, beginning in the late nineteenth century, involved how city councils across America began enacting ordinances, the vagrancy laws. The ordinances classified as a misdemeanor public appearance by facially different people. These city codes became known as the Ugly Laws.

City of Chicago Municipal Code, sec. 36034

"No person who is diseased, maimed, mutilated or in any way deformed so as to be an unsightly or disgusting object or improper person to be allowed in or on the public ways or other public places in this city, or shall therein or thereon expose himself to public view, under a penalty of not less than one dollar nor more than fifty dollars for each offense." (Repealed 1974).

Why did Hank at the meeting go off on the topic of ADA (the Americans with Disabilities Act)? Who knows for sure? I can say with certainty our "faces" are important. Our face is like "You Central." Think about all the people you have met in your life whom you identify only by their face. You see with your eyes, smell with your nose; hear with your ears, and on and on. When someone takes a photo of you, it is your face they want to photograph.

It's typical to find people wanting a face-to-face meeting. They want to read the person's facial expressions to understand what is going on beyond mere words. That is a sensible expectation, and that's key to successful communication. The essence of acting is learning all kinds of facial expressions. Our nature dictates this, a practice common to all from cradle to grave.

Several years ago, during one of the Super Bowls, a detergent company introduced a commercial. A guy with a stain on his shirt was interviewing for a job. The interviewer could only focus on the stain. That is what it is like to have a facial difference. I have had ten times more physical issues with swallowing, my hand shaking and my lack of mobility. As the detergent commercial illustrated, people expect the shirt to be clean. Because of my face being half paralyzed, my facial expressions are not what people expect. When I laugh, the muscles on the right side of my face work while the paralyzed muscles on the left side do nothing.

Besides my facial paralysis, the muscles that should help my jaw chew food exhibit acute atrophy and paralysis. My jaw muscles combined with my half paralyzed swallowing mechanism can make eating difficult. I have learned to put my bent index finger under my jaw, below my mouth, to help chew food. I have eaten this way for as long as I remember. In fact, it is second nature to me. Most of the time, I am not even aware I am doing it.

The world is what it is, like it or not, and some kids are going to tease other children about many things. Life goes on. I cannot imagine parenting a child who is different, regardless of why. I am very familiar with what it is like being the focus of unnecessary and unwanted attention.

There is little to nothing a parent can do to prevent a child from getting bullied by other children or, even worse, by adults, like my third grade elementary school teacher. Adults are the people you would think should know better, but some do not. When teasing or verbal abuse comes from adults, it is crueler and the sting lasts a lifetime.

In my experience, what makes matters worse is being the target of this abuse. Worse yet, is keeping the bullying to yourself, which I did.

As mean as some people were to me, polite avoidance, rather than other more extreme forms of bigotry, caused a slow, steady burn in my soul.

What kind of person responds to my facial difference by staring at me? Are they less educated? Are they crude, insensitive people who do not care about others' feelings? In my experience, it is something more fundamental to human nature to check out appearance different from our own? People of all races, creeds and nationalities showed me great kindness. Why do we concentrate on those who reject us?

I am a woodworker and a good one, if I do not say so myself! I would take part in fine art shows around the country. Hundreds upon hundreds of people would see my work and tell me how they admired the craftmanship in my work. That was nice and as a craftsman, I appreciated the compliment. Other woodworkers would tell me how they admired the craftsmanship. Everyone's positive comments gave me a great sense of satisfaction.

In the evening after the show, what did I obsess about? Not the hundreds of people who paid me a compliment, but the one or two people who did not like my work. Why do we do that to ourselves? The same is true with our facial differences. Most people put our differences aside and treat us as they would treat anyone else. Some people will react to your face, but the overwhelming majority will move on and want to get to know you as a person. They will treat you with respect and dignity.

The point is this; we cannot go through our lives being victims! If you want to improve your life, start with the person staring back at you in the mirror. The people, both good and bad, in this essay will always exist, and what they think and do will only matter if we give them permission.

You know better than to become a person who sprays a child down with a garden hose. Don't be the schoolteacher who, because of her messy personal life, abuses those who cannot fight back. Their actions were deliberate and directed at me, but it does not give me the right to hurt others. It's easy to get bitter and angry. It's much better to concentrate on myself and make sure I do not become the type of person I have grown to dislike.

If your life is anything like mine, you will discover this. Most individuals you encounter in your lifetime will possess a compassionate nature as they navigate their own personal challenges. Don't let those few people who judge you dominate how you view the world.

This essay is my story. How I lived with a facial difference. Many facially different people of my generation have, in our own way, tried to set an example for future generations. Younger generations are redefining beauty, decency, and what it means to participate in our society.

People are challenging long held institutional assumptions. People within organizations are forcing institutions around the globe to reevaluate long-held beliefs. How can we ignore the rights of others and expect equal rights for ourselves?

If you belong to a group that holds arcane beliefs, you need to reevaluate your priorities. Either help to change your organization's priorities and beliefs or leave the group. There is no place or justification for bigotry in our institutions, our government, or anywhere in our country.

A significant number of people in the United States and worldwide are without the advantages most people enjoy. Every day, these marginalized people put up with humiliating demoralizing treatment. I can tell you from firsthand experience it is exhausting being the focal point of unwarranted and unwanted bigotry.

Here's the truth: every day in America, police are pulling over Black and Latino people because of their color. Some fanatical religious groups have targeted the LGBTQ community. Thousands of people, for all kinds of reasons, are being denied basic human rights and full access to the benefits of our society.

As important as these issues are today, they will be much more important in the future. To tackle how we live in the future, we will require an all hands on deck approach.

We can no longer afford the philosophy that some people are less than others. We need everyone's participation to address unprecedented problems. Everyone, without exception, needs a seat at the table.

Tid bits

Polio has been my unwanted and unwelcome companion since July 5, 1951. Every day since, without exception, it has been part of my life.

People are baffling to me. I don't understand why some feel the need to stare when I'm in public. I've always wondered what's going on behind their penetrating eyes. What are they thinking? What do they think staring is going to do? I will never understand that aspect of our nature.

I have been the recipient of the kindest people you can imagine. Yet, because of my facial difference, I have been the target of the most spiteful, despicable people. How can one person see those of us who are different with such contempt and yet another with so much kindness and possibility? It is disheartening to realize that we all have so much to learn about kindness and treating one another with decency.

All I know with absolute certainty is that we all get old, and we all die. Our life spans are short, we must do the best we can with the short time we have. Like everyone on this planet, we are all a work in progress. As individuals, we must learn to put aside our own bigotries. As institutions, we can no longer use the scriptures as authorization to discriminate. We are all flawed, therefore all our institutions are flawed. The time is at hand to include everyone, to let everyone participate in the bounties of life. We are wasting so much of our potential and so much of our collective humanity.

Saying that polio is a terrible disease is an understatement. Unfortunately, it's only one of hundreds of chronic diseases and maladies that impact lives around the world. During the pandemic, vaccinations became a political hot topic. I'll be the first to admit, there is no such thing as the perfect vaccine. Automobiles are sometimes deadly, but that doesn't mean we have to stop driving. There is a risk versus reward equation in everything we do. It must be a mixture of arrogance, ignorance, and naivety that a person doesn't feel the need to not get vaccinated. The polio virus is one of hundreds of crippling viruses, not to mention all the other maladies that cause irreparable lifelong damage both physically and from a psychosocial point of reference. I wouldn't wish any of these life changing diseases on my worst enemy. In this essay, I listed a fraction of the things that happen to me throughout my life. The aftermath of these diseases can be and usually are pure unadulterated hell. If you are one of those who have yet to get vaccinated, PLEASE reconsider! You don't want to contract a crippling disease or worse yet inflict one of these terrible and preventable diseases on someone who is vulnerable. You don't have the right to do that. It is plain and simply cruel.

Regardless of what makes you different, be who you are, no matter what. Learn to like yourself just the way you are, regardless of what other people or institutions say or do.

Your Rights:
Strive to be happy. However, you define happiness.
Do your thing. Be whatever you want to be.
Be kind to yourself.
Chill out and live and let live. Show respect to others.
Live in the moment.

Your Obligations
The world is not and will never be a perfect place.
Be the best the best version of yourself.
Be kind. If you find it difficult, do it anyway.
Show love and respect to those who love you while quietly ignore others who don't.
Do not become a cynic, it is a waste of time.
Set an example for decency.
If a person or institution says you're not good enough...quietly and purposely leave!
To those who have a stake in making the world a better place:

There have been times during my life where I was the bad example, but I finally grew up. I was a troubled teenager with a big chip on my shoulder. During my sophomore year at Gilbert High School in 1965, my English teacher, Mrs. Pitts, asked me to stay after class. She wanted to talk to me. I was worried that I had done something wrong. To my surprise, she told me I had the potential to be an excellent writer. I was, to say the least, shocked. She encouraged me to enter a national wide short story contest. She offered her help as an editor in helping me become the best writer I could be. I'd never thought about writing. At that time in my life, I spent most of my time wallowing around in my crap. Mrs. Pitts, for whatever reason, planted a seed that is still vibrant after 60 years.

Like my father and my grandfather, I always been a woodworker. Both writing and working with wood have become the activities where I go to relax. When anyone learns a new discipline, there is an enormous of work that must happen before you produce work that is excellent, by any measure. This is true about woodworking or writing. I've never been the best writer when it comes to grammar, but thanks to a lot of expert advice from incredible editors in recent years, I'm putting out good writing, at least I think so! (Thank you, Dawn!)

I've strived to be an excellent writer and a good woodworker by any measure. I want to be the best I can be because of all the work I put into woodworking and writing my stories.

I leave you with these thoughts. Excluding people from having a seat at the table has always been and will forever be a bad idea. It is a belief whose time is long overdue to disappear. We are living in an era where old assumptions are being questioned. Are these assumptions still relevant? Were they ever relevant? Some of these ideas were the bedrock of our collective beliefs. Our world is struggling with dramatic changes never seen before in all human history.

People are redefining what it means to love another human being. The LGBT community has fought a long hard battle for equal rights. Gay and transgendered people have always been part of every society that ever existed anywhere. Recognizing their basic human rights is long overdue.

We must demand basic human rights for all people, regardless of how society defines them. This new way of thinking has pressured religious institutions around the world. The argument used today by religions to oppose gay marriage is nothing new. Sixty years ago, various religions used the same argument against interracial marriage.

I wrote this essay for the people all around the world who are just like me. We are odd ones, the social misfits who, for a variety of reasons, do not fit in. The ones who are different like me, those of us who feel like the square peg in a round hole.

This essay is short by design. A non-reader can read the book in one sitting. It is also my recollection of events that happened over my lifetime. I thought long and hard about the people I want to reach. What stories should I include? In the end, I shared the stories that had the most impact on my life. I choose to challenge long-held beliefs by many institutions that discourage inclusion.

I'm compelled to keep saying that our country, like all countries around the world, is full of instances when we didn't act for the common good. Not that long ago that city councils enacted the "ugly" laws and "sundown" laws. Laws that targeted disabled/disfigured people and minorities by restricting their movement. We can dress up our bigotry as a city ordinance, religious dogma, or political rhetoric, but in the end it's just plain old in your face bigotry. How can we have any expectation of change if we hold bigoted ideas about who gets to have full access as a human being? At the root of these stories are people's misconceptions about those of us who are different.

There are a few things I have learned along the way. I'm an old man who has lived with a facial disfigurement for most of my life. People have gawked at me, gossiped about me, refused to wait on me in some restaurants. People have marginalized, mocked, marginalized, outcast, and bullied me, only because my face looks different. I can tell you as one who has been receiving this bigotry, it is not fun, not the least little bit.

Excuse me?

Things people said to me over the years. Please note these little tid bits happened. I obviously took a literary license because I remember the conversations but note all the circumstances.

Richfield Gas Station ~ Gilbert, Arizona circa 1959
"What happened?"
"I'm sorry?"
"Your face, what happened?"
"I had Polio."
"No, you're too young."
"That's what my parents told me,"
"No, it's genetic."

Safeway ~ Indianapolis, Indiana circa 1994
"Hi," said a little boy sitting in the seat of his father's grocery cart.
"Hello back to you. How are you today young man?"
The kid noticed my facial difference. "Dad what happened to the man standing by me?"

The father a skinny thirty something, long hair guy, with tattoos all over, turned around to see what his son was talking about. He smiled at me then asked, "What did you asked?"

"What happened to that man's face," pointing at me.

I smiled, subtilling telling the boy's father that his son's question was an innocent gesture.

The tattooed father paused for a couple of seconds and replied, "I have no idea what happened to his face. If you really need to know, ask him he's standing right behind you."

The little boy asked, and I answered. Many people would have been upset at their child for asking such a personal inappropriate question. The quick acting father decided to make this embarrassing situation a teaching moment. The little was curious not trying to be mean. Life goes on.

Maricopa County ~ 1968 - Yavapai, County ~ 1971

"Do you have you license and registration?"

"Yeah, here you go."

"How much have you had to drink tonight?"

"If you're talking about alcohol, none."

"Why are you slurring your words?"

"I had polio as a kid."

"Oh yeah, my sister had polio her speech is okay."

Capital Feed and Seed ~ Gilbert, Arizona circa 1960

"I heard you got the polio."

"Yes sir."

"Is that what screwed up your face?"

"Well...Yes sir I guess."

"Who told you THAT?"

"Who told me what?"

"That you had some kind of special face polio?"

"My Mom and Dad. Why?"
"Noth'n just thought I'd ask."

Jake's Good Eats Dairy Bar ~ Gilbert, Arizona circa 1972
"Ball's Palsy?"
"You mean Bell's Palsy."
"Yeah, whatever."
"What? Do you want to know if I have it?"
"Yeah."
"No. I had polio."
"You got polio of the face? Are you messing with me?"

Burger King ~ Kansas City ~ circa 1982
"Man...that has to hurt?"
"Pardon me?"
"You were at the dentist, right? It looks like he just beat the crap out of you. Does it hurt?
"No, I'm fine."

Wichita, Kansas ~ circa 1989
"Do you have your driver's license, registration and insurance card?"
"I sure do officer, here you go."
"How much have you had to drink tonight?"
"If you're talking about alcohol, none."
"Why are you slurring your words?"
"I had polio as a kid."
"Would you mind getting out of the car?

Urgent Care ~ Phoenix circa ~ 2006
"Oh my God, what happened?"
"I have the worst cold than I've had in years."
"A cold did that to your face?"
"What?"
"What caused your face to look that way?"

"Are you a doctor? I came here because I have an awful cold. I had polio that's what happened to my face."

"You had face polio? Wow! I never heard of that!"

"Are you a doctor?"

Home Depot–Phoenix, Arizona

"Stroke?"

"I beg your pardon?"

"When did you have the stroke?"

"I didn't have a stroke."

"So, I don't get it, what happened?"

"What's going on? Are you writing a book?"

"Screw you, I was just trying to be nice

My Grandfather's shop

My essay ends in my grandfather's woodworking shop in June 1967. During my recovery from jaw surgery, I visited my grandparents' home in Prescott, Arizona. As usual, the aftermath of the surgery left me an emotional wreck. My whole body hurt, and my jaw was wired shut. Everything I ate had to work its way through a straw. It's an excellent way to lose weight.

My grandfather and I were in his woodworking shop when, surprisingly, he inquired, "What are you going to do when you grow up?"

"I don't know."

He paused and said, "You're a creative kid. Why not study to become a writer or a comedian? Your quick and have an uncanny ability to make people laugh."

"Oh yeah?"

"The truth is you'd be good at whatever you decide you want to do with your life."

While I appreciated his kind words, I sensed it was a caring, yet empty, gesture. I was recovering from major surgery and a long stay in Phoenix Crippled Children's Hospital. I entered the fourth year of my facial reconstruction. It seemed like a perpetual list of never rending procedures and operations that left me drained.

My depression highlighted the disbelief in my grandfather's story. Only after living most of my life did, I realize the depth of his sincerity and decency.

"I enjoy writing stories," I told my grandfather after some reflection.

"Good for you," he said, resuming his work. Someday, when you're an old man like me, you should write about your experiences. Help people understand your life experiences.

Honor those who helped you along the way. I believe you would excel at assisting others in comprehending your life experiences.

"Yeah Grandpa, someday I'll do that."

"I'm serious," he said. "Write your story, it's important."

Fifty-seven years later, I told my story as I promised my grandfather.

The understanding that we all possess much to learn about kindness and decent treatment of each other is disheartening. My only certainty regarding life is that it is not a dress rehearsal. Life is short. We must do the best we can with what we have. Like everyone on this planet, we are all a work in progress. As individuals, we must learn to put aside our bigotry. All people, including you and me, are flawed.

All of us have terrible pain tucked away, staying rent free in our personal thoughts. Don't let those secret, hurtful thoughts occupy your mind. You're in charge, express your pain in your music, your art, or like I try to do in my writing. We aren't warehouses to store all the nasty things that have happened throughout our lives. Tell them time is up and kick them out of your thoughts and heal.

Addendum

"A hidden community: Facial disfigurement as a globally neglected human rights issue." by Phyllida Swift and Kathleen Bogart

This abstract was first published by the Journal of Oral Biology and Craniofacial Research in September 2021. It is one of the best academic papers published on this subject. I encourage to take a few minutes and read this abstract.

A hidden community: Facial disfigurement as a globally neglected human rights issue, follows a clear structure: introduction, background on Face Equality International, the importance of language, wellbeing needs, social and societal barriers (with case studies), attitudes towards facial disfigurement, disfigurement as a hidden human rights issue, the legal context, and conclusion.

The introduction highlights the gap in disability rights concerning disfigurement and outlining the abstract's purpose. The conclusion provides a strong summary and reiterates the call for action, bringing the discussion to a close.

This abstract presents a compelling case for increased attention to the rights and needs of individuals with facial disfigurements. The abstract's

strong arguments, well-structured organization, and impactful case studies make it a valuable contribution to the field.
https://pmc.ncbi.nlm.nih.gov/articles/PMC8476770/
Google search: A hidden community: Facial disfigurement as a globally neglected human rights issue
Contact Information for the authors:
Phyllida Swift, Email: phyllida.swift@faceequalityinternational.org.
Kathleen Bogart, Email: kathleen.bogart@oregonstate.edu.

Books about, The History of Disabilities
Helen Keller: Selected Writings by Kim E. Nielson 2005
The Ugly Laws: Disability in Public by Susan M. Schwelk 2009
Words Made Flesh: Nineteenth-Century Deaf Education and the Growth of Deaf Culture 2012
The New Disability History: American Perspectives 2001
Psychosocial Aspects of Health Care: by Meredith Drench, Ann Noonan, Nancy Sharby, and Susan Ventura 2011

FACES: The National Craniofacial Association
FACES: has a comprehensive list of worldwide Support Groups, Camps and Retreats, and Educational Scholarships. This world class organization offers all kinds of help, not to mention Public Awareness, Understanding, Information, and Support.
5325 Old Hixson Pike – Hixson, TN 37343
Phone: 1 (423) 266 1632 Toll Free 1 800 332-2373
Link to their website: https://www.faces-cranio.org/services
FACES: The National Craniofacial Association is a non-profit organization serving children and adults throughout the United States with severe craniofacial differences resulting from birth defects, injuries, or disease. There is never a charge for any service provided by FACES.

Adults Facial Differences Community on Facebook: Adults Facial Difference Community Facebook support for adults with a facial difference.

How to contact the author:

m.e. Mark Elzey
(520) 465-6378
elzey@me.com

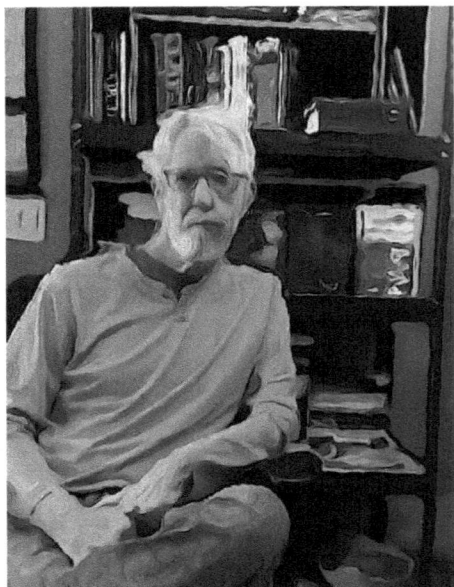

About the Author

We are all ultimately defined by the events in our lives I'm no exception. The first defining experience in my life was contracting Bulbar Polio at eighteen months of age. My second experience was being raised in Gilbert, Arizona, during the fifties and sixties. It was an idyllic Southwest community of mid-twentieth century American. The population was around 1800 people, including those who lived outside the city limits.

My wife (also a Gilbert girl) live in Marana, Arizona, a northwestern suburb of Tucson. She's also my best friend, my squeeze, doubles as my editor, and is my most ardent fan and my most vocal critique.

www.ingramcontent.com/pod-product-compliance
Lightning Source LLC
Chambersburg PA
CBHW060521280326
41933CB00014B/3054